I0439467

**TABLE OF CONTENTS**

**Anti Aging Techniques EXPOSED Vol 6**
The Anti-aging Lifestyle: 10 Simple Steps to Turn Back the Clock
©Copyright 2013 by Dr. Noah Pranksky

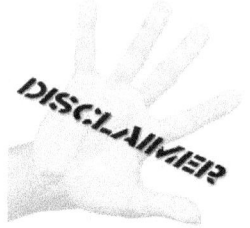

## DISCLAIMER AND TERMS OF USE AGREEMENT:

**(Please Read This Before Using This Book)**

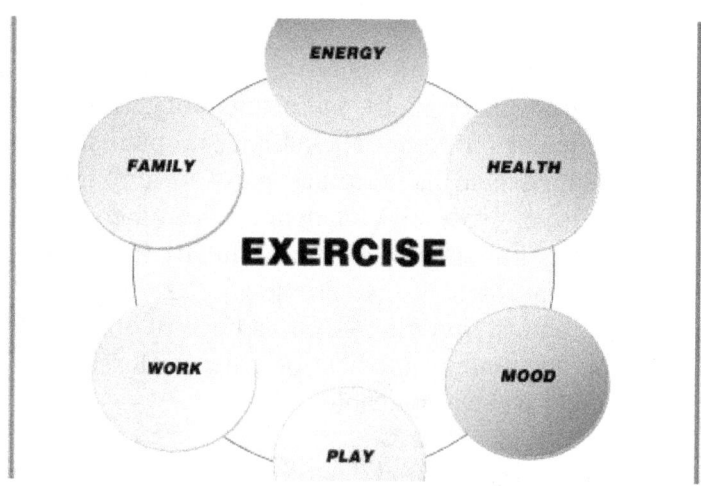

A lifestyle is made up of various habits. All people respond, to various stimuli, based on how they are trained. Over the years, people have learned to react to certain situations with a predictable behavioral pattern. Habits through practice turn into behavior - both good and bad. Like I said, not all habits are good habits either. A person suffers from his/her own personal problems, like you, and the stress and anxiety his/her choices bring. Wrongful choices evoke stress and anxiety. This is important to understand completely. Wrongful choices evoke suffering. This suffering takes the form of anxiety, stress, and other psychosomatic ailments.

My whole goal of this 6-volumes series on Anti-Aging has been to make you aware of your present lifestyle and how certain changes with retard the aging process and give you a better quality of life.

This is the sixth and final book in the Anti-Aging series. I hope you enjoyed my efforts. Now I want to pull it all together and go out with a BANG!

**This Lifestyles Regimen Program involves the following supplements:**

**Natural Organic Oils** (1,000 mgs gel caps recommended) made from a variety of natural oils such as flaxseed, sesame, sunflower, etc. containing:

- Alpha-Linolenic Acid/Omega-3
- Linoleic Acid/Omega-6
- Oleic Acid/Omega-9

Any health food store carries flaxseed oil gel caps. Make sure, by reading the label on the bottle that it is 1,000 mgs, that it contains the three above Omega 3, 6, 9 ingredients. Also, keep the open bottle refrigerated.

**Directions: take 3-capsules in the morning 30-minutes before eating and 3-capsules in the evening 30-minutes before eating.**

**Comprehensive Mineral Supplement** (amino acid chelated) containing the following nine essential minerals: boron, iron, magnesium, zinc, selenium, copper, manganese, chromium, potassium, as well as containing the following key ingredients: molybdenum, l-glutamic acid, MSM (methylsulfonylmethane), horsetail extract, sulfer, vanadium, phosphorus, and calcium. Make sure the mineral supplement is amino acid chelated!!! If it is not, you are wasting your money.

5

Furthermore, make sure it contains the above nine essential minerals. The word "essential" means that they are not obtained in your diet and are needed as a supplement.

**Directions:  Take two (2) tablets daily.**

**Detoxification Tea** containing the following certified organic ingredients:  burdock root, sheep sorrel herb, slippery elm bark, watercress herb, Turkish rhubarb root, blessed thistle herb, and red clover blossom.  Use a tea that is an Esiac formulation and is of superior quality.

**Directions:   Follow manufacturer's instructions to make tea as well as dosage amount.**

**HGH Supplement:** an amino acid based precursor that causes the pituitary gland to secrete more human growth hormone.

**Directions:  Follow manufacturer's instructions.**

- Limit ingestion of carbohydrates to 20% of a total dietary intake of 2,000 calories/day.  1 gram of carbs =1tsp. of sugar = 5 calories.
- Light exercise (anaerobic is preferred) is recommended.

## Chapter 1 - Live Longer, Have Fun

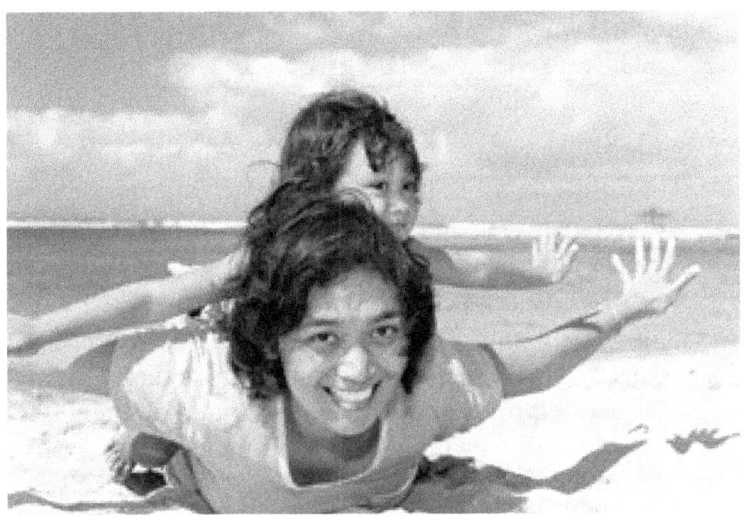

A healthy lifestyle doesn't have to mean treadmills and salads every day. Many activities that are fun and pleasurable are also good for you. By understanding how these activities can help you live longer and what to do to get the most benefits, you'll be putting some fun into healthy living.

### 1. Drink Red Wine

Red wine is packed with resveratrol, an antioxidant. These work to protect your body against the effects of aging. One or 2 glasses of red wine a day can help keep your body young.

### 2. Eat Dark Chocolate

Dark chocolate is a wonderful food that contains a large amount of antioxidants that protect your body from aging. Find good quality dark chocolate, learn to appreciate it, and have a bit of it each day. Eating chocolate may lower your blood pressure and cholesterol while providing an energy boost.

### 3. Smile

Smiling is a great way to change your attitude, connect with people and give benefit to your body. Like relaxation, smiling can work to counteract the effects of stress. By forcing ourselves to smile, we "trick" our body into believing that everything is good, thereby reducing stress. Like a switch, smiling can actually change your mood. So put a smile on, even if you don't feel like it, and pretty soon you'll be smiling for real.

### 4. Have More Sex

Sex and touching are thought to be essential parts of health. Sex releases an assortment of beneficial chemicals in the body. Sex and touching help us bond with others, strengthen relationships, and increase our own self-worth. Frequent sex may even extend your life by years.

### 5. Relax

Relaxation is the opposite of stress. While stress brings harmful health effects, relaxation helps our bodies to rest, heal and function better. By practicing daily relaxation techniques, you can train yourself to turn off your stress and replace it with calm energy. This will improve your blood pressure, heart rate and ability to cope with life's challenges.

### 6. Make Exercise Play

Physical games and sports are a great way to keep both your body and mind healthy. Simple exercise routines are great for maintaining balance, flexibility, endurance and strength. Group games and sports can give your mind a workout as well, as you anticipate other people's actions and how to work together. Find a game and activity that suits your level of physical ability and play often.

## 7. Sleep

Sleep is an essential body function. Most Americans do not get enough sleep. Medications, stress, illness and poor sleep habits all can prevent you from getting between 7 and 9 hours a night. The health benefits of sleep include more energy, better immune function, and more.

## 8. Spend Time With Loved Ones

Relationships are an important part of health. Not only do strong bonds with other people mean you will have help when you need it, being connected also means protection from loneliness, depression, and mental illness. Spend time cultivating your relationships with friends and family to improve your health and your life.

## 9. Solve Puzzles and Play Brain Games

Mind games are a great way to stay involved and engaged in the world. Games can exercise different parts of your mind and entice your curiosity. If possible, choose social games like chess or bridge that exercise your brain while keeping you connected with others.

## 10. Be Positive

Having a positive attitude about aging can add more than seven years to your life, according to researchers. Avoid the cultural push to glorify youth and regret each passing year. Find ways to pleasure in your increasing age and enjoy greater learning, experience, and control in your life.

**Play Games, Age Well**

Brain fitness has basic principles: variety and curiosity. When anything you do becomes second nature, you need to make a change. If you can do the crossword puzzle in your sleep, it's time for you to move on to a new challenge in order to get the best workout for your brain. Curiosity about the world around you, how it works and how you can understand it will keep your brain working fast and efficiently. Use the ideas below to help attain your quest for mental fitness.

**1. Play Games**

Brain fitness programs and games are a wonderful way to tease and challenge your brain. Suduko, crosswords and electronic games can all improve your brain's speed and memory. These games rely on logic, word skills, math and more. These games are also fun. You'll get benefit more by doing these games a little bit every day -- spend 15 minutes or so, not hours.

**2. Meditation**

Daily meditation is perhaps the single greatest thing you can do for your mind/body health. Meditation not only relaxes you, it gives your brain a workout. By creating a different mental state, you engage your brain in new and interesting ways while increasing your brain fitness.

### 3. Eat for Your Brain

Your brain needs you to eat healthy fats. Focus on fish oils from wild salmon, nuts such as walnuts, seeds such as flax seed and olive oil. Eat more of these foods and less saturated fats. Eliminate trans fats completely from your diet.

### 4. Tell Good Stories

Stories are a way that we solidify memories, interpret events and share moments. Practice telling your stories, both new and old, so that they are interesting, compelling and fun. Some basic storytelling techniques will go a long way in keeping people's interest both in you and in what you have to say.

### 5. Turn Off Your Television

The average person watches more than 4 hours of television every day. Television can stand in the way of relationships, life and more. Turn off your TV and spend more time living and exercising your mind and body.

### 6. Exercise Your Body To Exercise Your Brain

Physical exercise is great brain exercise too. By moving your body, your brain has to learn new muscle skills, estimate distance and practice balance. Choose a variety of exercises to challenge your brain.

### 7. Read Something Different

Books are portable, free from libraries and filled with infinite interesting characters, information and facts. Branch out from familiar reading topics. If you usually read history books, try a contemporary novel. Read foreign authors, the classics and random books. Not only will your brain get a workout by imagining different time periods, cultures and peoples, you will also have interesting stories to tell about your reading, what it makes you think of and the connections you draw between modern life and the words.

### 8. Learn a New Skill

Learning a new skill works multiple areas of the brain. Your memory comes into play, you learn new movements and you associate things differently. Reading Shakespeare, learning to cook and building an airplane out of toothpicks all will challenge your brain and give you something to think about.

### 9. Make Simple Changes

We love our routines. We have hobbies and pastimes that we could do for hours on end. But the more something is 'second nature,' the less our brains have to work to do it. To really help your brain stay young, challenge it. Change routes to the grocery store, use your opposite hand to open doors and eat dessert first. All this will force your brain to wake up from habits and pay attention again.

### 10. Train Your Brain

Brain training is becoming a trend. There are formal courses, websites and books with programs on how to train your brain to work better and faster. There is some research behind these programs, but the basic principles are memory, visualization and reasoning. Work on these three concepts everyday and your brain will be ready for anything.

## Chapter 2 - More Sex, Live longer

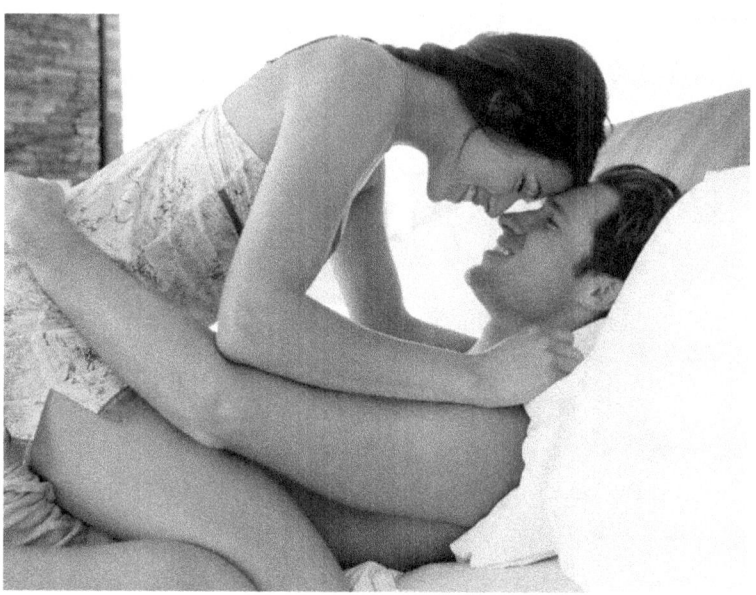

## Women, Aging and Sex

Sex and aging are topics most older women do not want to talk about. The most obvious changes in a woman's body as she ages come with menopause. During menopause, decreasing estrogen levels cause physical changes that may impact sexual function. Aging may also bring emotions that can interfere with sex (see these sex tips for the older women for some help).

## Menopause and Decrease in Estrogen

During menopause, the levels of estrogen are reduced. These estrogen decreases alter the thickness and size of a woman's reproductive organs. These changes include:

- Loss of elasticity and a thinning of the vaginal tissue
- Decrease in the amount of lubrication
- Decrease in the size of the clitoral, vulvar and labial tissues
- Decreases in the size of the cervix, uterus and ovaries

### The Impact on Sex

These changes alter the experience of sex in the following ways:

- The anticipation before orgasm decreases
- Orgasms may be less intense
- Sexual desire may be reduced
- However, the sensitivity of the clitoris remains the same

### Medical Procedures and Sexual Desire

Emotions can impact both sexual desire and sexual satisfaction. As women age, the changes in their bodies can trigger powerful emotions. Surgical procedures can also change how a woman feels about her own body. Some examples of how aging impacts sex through emotions includes:

- **Hysterectomy (removal of the uterus and sometimes ovaries):** This surgical procedure does not change a woman's ability to have sex, though both strong emotions about this procedure and changes in hormones can impact sexual desire.

- **Mastectomy (removal of a breast due to cancer):** A mastectomy can radically alter how a woman perceives her own beauty and sexual attractiveness. Open communication with your sexual partner can help tremendously.

## Health Conditions and Sexual Function

Many chronic health conditions can interfere with sex. Conditions such as arthritis can make sex painful. Heart disease can make the physical activity of sex difficult. By aggressively managing your health conditions, you can improve the quality of your sexual experiences.

## Perception of Aging

How women perceive themselves as they age greatly impacts sexual desire. In our culture, we are constantly exposed to images of youth. As we age, there is little to reassure women that they are still sexually attractive and beautiful.

Because of this, women may lose interest in sex as they age. Talking about these emotions with your sexual partner can help relieve some of the stress around body image and aging.

## Men, Aging and Sex

Primarily due to a drop in testosterone, men will experience changes in their sexual function as they age.

These changes include (see sex tips for the older man for tips on dealing with these changes):

- Fewer sperm are produced
- Erections take longer to occur
- Erections may not be as hard
- The 'recovery time' (time between erections) increases to 12 to 24 hours
- The force of ejaculation decreases
- Sexual desire decreases are due to emotional reasons or health problems

### Decreased Testosterone

As a man ages, his testosterone levels decrease. Typically this decrease in testosterone stabilizes around age 60. Testosterone decrease is the primary reason for many of the conditions listed above. Testosterone replacement therapy is becoming popular for addressing concerns of aging men. This type of hormone treatment is controversial and should be approached with caution. Increasing muscle mass through exercise and proper nutrition can help maintain a healthy testosterone level.

### Cardiovascular Disease, High Blood Pressure and Male Sexual Health

These health conditions alter how the blood flows in the body. When the arteries become narrower and harder, blood does not flow as freely. This can be troublesome for men trying to achieve an erection, as erections depend on the ability of blood to fill the penis. Controlling high blood pressure and other cardiovascular diseases through lifestyle change and medication can improve sexual performance.

**Diabetes and Male Sexual Health**

Many men with diabetes have normal sexual lives. However, diabetes can cause impotence, the inability to have sex. Men with diabetes are approximately three times more likely to experience erectile dysfunction than men without diabetes. They also experience this condition approximately 15 years earlier than men without diabetes. If you have diabetes and are having trouble maintaining an erection, talk to your doctor. Many medications can help.

**Pain and Male Sexual Health**

Many health conditions such as arthritis, back pain and shingles can interfere with sex by causing pain that may make sex uncomfortable. These conditions also can alter your mood, sleep habits and attitudes. Experimenting with different sexual positions and techniques can help. You can also talk with your doctor about managing pain.

**Incontinence and Male Sexual Health**

Incontinence is the loss of bladder control which can cause urine leakage. This condition becomes more common as people age. Often leakage occurs during exercise, laughing or coughing. During sex, extra pressure is placed on your bladder. Men with an incontinence condition may be afraid to have sex. By controlling incontinence through medical or behavioral approaches, the chance of leakage during sex can be greatly reduced.

**Medications and Male Sexual Health**

Some of the medications prescribed to treat common age-related health conditions can interfere with sex. Some blood pressure medicines, antidepressants and diabetes drugs can make it more difficult for men to maintain an erection. These medications can also reduce sexual desire. You may be able to use alternative medications if you experience these side effects. Talk to your doctor.

**Prostatectomy: Prostate Surgery**

A prostatectomy is a surgical procedure that removes some or all of a man's prostate. This is often done to treat prostate cancer or an enlarged prostate. A consequence of this surgery can be incontinence or impotence. Before undergoing a prostatectomy, be sure to talk to your doctor

If you are not satisfied with your sexual ability, talk to doctor. Changes in your medication, managing your health conditions and treatment of sexual problems may help.

**Sex Tips for Older Women**

Your sex life will change as your body ages. These changes can be addressed and you can have healthy, satisfying sex your entire life. By communicating with your partner, taking care of your health and maintaining a good emotional perspective, your sex life can grow richer with the years.

**1. Talk With Your Partner**

Open communication has always been essential for good sex. Talk with your partner about any sexual difficulties you might be having as a couple. Try to treat the difficulties as problems to solve and work together on finding creative solutions.

## 2. Lubricate

As a woman ages, natural lubrication for sexual intercourse decreases. This is easily fixed by using a water-based lubricant. At first, applying a lubricant for sex may seem awkward, but you and your partner will quickly become used to it and can even incorporate it into foreplay.

## 3. Experiment with Positions and Times

Pain caused by arthritis or other condition can interfere with sex. Experiment with different sexual positions, and you may find one that works much better. Also, arthritis and other pain conditions are often less severe at certain times a day, which will vary for each person. Try having sex when your pain is the least severe.

## 4. Deal with Erectile Problems

For men, trouble having an erection is an expected part of aging. If this happens to your partner, gently help him troubleshoot this problem. Lifestyle changes and medications that can help.

## 5. Feel Beautiful

We live in a culture that is constantly showing us images of youth and beauty. As women age, they may feel less sexually attractive, which can interfere with sexual desire. Try not to be influenced by these cultural messages. Sure, your body changes as you age, but that does not reflect on your worth or desirability. Ignore messages and stereotypes from television, magazines and other media sources and embrace your body at every stage of your life.

### 6. Take Care of Your Health

Poor health can interfere with sexual satisfaction. If you have a health condition, be sure to the manage it. Follow your doctor's orders and make the lifestyle changes you need to be healthy. Losing weight, exercising and eating well will not only improve your health, your sex life will also improve.

### 7. Sex After Surgery

As women age, they may need to undergo surgical procedures that alter the reproductive organs. The most common are mastectomy (the removal of a breast or part of a breast to treat cancer) or hysterectomy (the removal of the uterus and sometimes the ovaries). These surgeries do not interfere with a woman's ability to have sex. However, these procedures can dramatically change how a woman perceives her own attractiveness. Open communication with your partner both before and after these procedures can help reduce anxiety and negativity.

### 8. Safe Sex

Any sexually active adult needs to protect herself from sexually transmitted diseases. Sexually transmitted infections, including HIV, are on the rise in older adults. Older adults have had more time to develop a sexual history. Also, many infections can remain dormant for years in people. Do not assume that an older sexual partner is a safe sexual partner. Always practice safe sex.

### 9. Talk to Your Doctor

If you or your partner is having sexual difficulties, talk to your doctor. There may be simple solutions to your problems such as changing the time of day that you take a medication or making lifestyle changes.

Expect that you will have to make adjustments in your life and sexual habits as you age. Your doctor can help your these adaptations go smoothly.

### 10. Vibrators and Masturbation

It is a simple fact that men have shorter life expectancies than women, resulting in a large number of older widowed or single women.

Sex and orgasms bring both emotional and physical benefits. Women should not feel guilty about masturbation. Vibrators and other devices can help tremendously.

### Sex Tips for Older Men

Maintaining your sexual health is an important part of aging. By keeping yourself healthy, confronting problems calmly and talking openly with your partner, you can improve your chances of having a long healthy sex life.

### 1. Talk Openly With Your Partner

Good sex always relies on open communication with your partner. As both of you age, things will change. These changes will require patience, understanding and experimentation. Emotions can greatly impact sexual health. By maintaining good communication and intimacy, you and your partner will be able to adapt to changes as necessary.

## 2. Manage Your Health Conditions

Health conditions like high blood pressure and chronic pain can make a healthy sex life difficult. By aggressively managing any health conditions, you can greatly reduce their impact on your sex life. A good approach is to follow your doctor's advice and make lifestyle changes.

## 3. Talk To Your Doctor

Your doctor cannot help you with your sexual concerns unless you mention them. Some sexual problems are actually medication side effects, which can be handled by adjusting medications that you are already taking or changing the time of day that you take medications. Many medications also directly treat sexual problems.

## 4. Experiment With Positions and Times

Sometimes changing the time of day or the position used in sex can relieve sexual problems. If a health condition is interfering with your sex life, you may notice that your symptoms are better at a certain time of day. Try having sex then. Varying the sexual positions that you use can help too, especially if pain from arthritis or other condition interferes with sex.

## 5. Expand Your Concept of Sex

Men tend to think of sex in terms of orgasms, but there can be a lot more to sex. As you age, you will need more time and physical contact to become aroused. Hugging, kissing and other forms of contact are essential parts of your sex life. If you find yourself living alone, masturbation can be part of a normal, healthy sex life.

## 6. Avoid Alcohol and Smoking

Both alcohol and smoking can hinder a man's ability to achieve an erection. These two substances alter the blood flow in your body and can limit the amount of blood that enters the penis. This can lead to the inability to have an erection, difficulty maintaining an erection or an erection that is softer than normal. If you are having sexual difficulties, consider abstaining from smoking and alcohol.

## 7. Expect Difficulties

As you age, you will experience certain changes in your sexual function. When these changes occur, don't panic. Rather, think of them as problems to be solved. If you react emotionally to these problems, you can make them worse. By expecting some degree of sexual change as you age, you can react calmly and troubleshoot your situation.

## 8. Eat Healthy and Lose Weight

Being overweight puts a strain on your body that can result in high blood pressure, heart disease, diabetes and other health conditions, all of which can interfere with a normal sex life. By eating healthy foods and losing excess weight you can prevent sexual problems.

## 9. Stay Sexually Active

If you have a long period of time in your life when you are sexually inactive, it will be more difficult to become sexually active later. Not only can frequent sex improve your sexual performance, it may even help you live longer.

### 10. Safe Sex

As more and more older people continue to have an active sex life, the issue of safe sex arises. All sexually active people must take this matter very seriously. STDs and HIV are on the rise in older adults. You cannot assume that having sex is risk-free just because you and your partner are older. In fact, as the age of your sexual partner increases, his or her sexual history is longer, too. Always practice safe sex.

### Brain Fitness

Happiness and aging are related, but not in the obvious way. We assume that our culture is a youth culture and that the young and the beautiful are the happiest people. That's just not true. The stereotype that young people are happy is just plain wrong. In fact, as a person ages, his or her chances at happiness only increase.

### Aging and Happiness

It is probably unfathomable for young people to think that their grandma or grandpa is happier than they are, but solid research shows that Americans get happier as they age. I love the fact that as I age I can look forward to more happiness, even despite any health conditions or other problems that may arise. Before we celebrate, though, let's take a good, hard look at the evidence on aging and happiness.

**Trends in Happiness Over Time**
Let's face it; research in to happiness is filled with judgments and subjectivity. How do I know that someone who says, "I'm pretty happy," on a survey really is? Maybe they just learned in their life to be content with less? Maybe they don't know what real happiness is? Maybe each generation has different expectations of happiness? Researchers had to figure a way around these types of problems.

Luckily, since 1972 sociologists have been surveying over 50,000 interviews in something called the "General Social Survey." Researchers can add questions, and questions are repeated for decades. The survey is open to the public (you can analyze the data yourself online). It is the source of lots of information about our society and perfect for a study on happiness over time. By comparing differently aged individuals over time within the same year, researchers were able to get around some of these problems. What they found is that happiness increases with age.

**Are You, In General, Very Happy, Pretty Happy or Not Too Happy?**
That is the big question they asked year after year while collecting data about the age of the people who answered. Not only were older people happier, the researchers found that this happiness was not something they had all

their life. In other words, when they got older (say 50+), happiness came to them.

**Aging America - A Happy Place**

So as the politicians and news media continue to warn us about the dangers of an aging America, keep this in mind: An aging America may be the happiest America we have ever seen. Perhaps this is because of the wisdom of years, perhaps older people adjust their expectations in life — but whatever the reason — there is good evidence through the study above (and others) that older Americans are truly happier than younger ones.

**More on Happy Aging**

To maximize your happiness as you age, try to ignore what you see in the culture about youth and happiness. Allow yourself to feel happy as you age and don't get caught up in worrying and fretting over things. Of course, take good care of your health and, most importantly, let yourself go a bit. Don't think that you have to act your age.

**Blood Pressure and Brain Aging**

High blood pressure (hypertension) is a common age-related health condition. When you blood pressure increases, it is hard on your heart and on your arteries. Turns out that high blood pressure can damage your brain as well, and not just from an increased risk of stroke.

People aged 60 and over with high blood pressure have a higher rate of cognitive decline and a greater risk of Alzheimer's disease than people with normal blood pressure. Using data from a national health survey, doctors discovered that men and women with healthy blood pressure showed the least amount of cognitive decline over time. Here are the numbers:

- For people aged 60 to 69, a blood pressure of 120.80 mmHg did best.
- For people aged 75 to 79, people under 140/90 mmHg had the best cognitive function.
- For people 80 or over, moderate high blood pressure was best.

As you age, it is likely that you blood pressure will increase. Making that increase as small as possible will protect both your heart and your brain. If you have high blood pressure, be sure to aggressively manage it through a combination of lifestyle changes like healthy eating and relaxation along with medication when suggested by a doctor. Keeping your blood pressure in normal ranges will slow your brain's aging.

**Alcohol and Your Brain**

For a while now, we have been hearing that drinking moderately can help improve your life expectancy and longevity. It does this by helping to protect your heart. But what if alcohol also protected your brain? Turns out that a moderate amount of daily alcohol does just that. Alcohol can protect your brain, your mental health and your cognitive (thinking) abilities.

Research shows that drinking moderately is better for you than drinking heavily or not drinking at all. Aim for around 2 servings of an alcoholic beverage a night (a serving is one glass of wine, one beer, one shot). Red wine is probably the best choice, as it has properties unrelated to alcohol that help slow aging.

British researchers, whose findings were published in a 2007 issue of the journal *Age and Ageing*, were interested in exploring whether alcohol consumption improved mental and cognitive health. They examined over 6,000 people over the age of 50. These people were part of a large-scale study on aging. They were asked questions about their alcohol consumption and were grouped into three categories for analysis: consumption of one or fewer drinks per day, 2 or fewer drinks per day and more than two drinks per day. The researchers also examined the participants' cognitive abilities, well-being and signs of depression.

Men and women in the 2 or fewer drinks per day group had better results for cognitive function, fewer signs of depression and a better sense of well-being. So go ahead and have 1 or 2 drinks a day if you want – do it for your heart, and do it for your brain. Remember, however, not to overdo it -- and that alcohol can pack a good amount of calories.

**Train Your Brain**

Memory is one of the most important skills of the brain. Having a good memory is a matter of making connections. The more connections you make around an item, the more likely you are to remember it.

Work on your memory by making as many connections as you can. If you want to remember a word, think about what other words sound the same, what that word makes you think of, and details about what you were doing when you heard the word. To remember a date, add the numbers together, multiply them or think of other things that happened on the same date. The key to exercising your memory is making connections.

## Visualization:

Visualizing is a great way to give your brain a workout. Pick a specific memory. Recall everything you can about it. Think about smells, what you were wearing, what you were thinking about. Say you want to visualize a beach vacation:

- picture the sand
- the feel of the sun
- the smell of sunscreen
- how you felt (tired, excited, relaxed?).

Think about who you traveled with, who you met there, and what you did.

Spend at least 15 minutes just visualizing everything. This exercises almost all functions of the brain: smells, sounds, tastes and sights. Repeat daily (with different memories) for a great brain fitness routine.

## Reasoning:

Reasoning is an important function of the brain that needs exercise to work well. Practice reasoning by asking the question "Why?". Why did the city begin the street repairs at the curb lane? Why do stores love to sell gift cards? Why are onions usually sautéed first, by themselves?

Just thinking about the possible answers to these questions will force your brain to use logic and intuition. Be curious about the world around you and ask yourself "Why?" all day long.

You will soon become good at finding the answers.

## Chapter 3 - Stress Relaxation

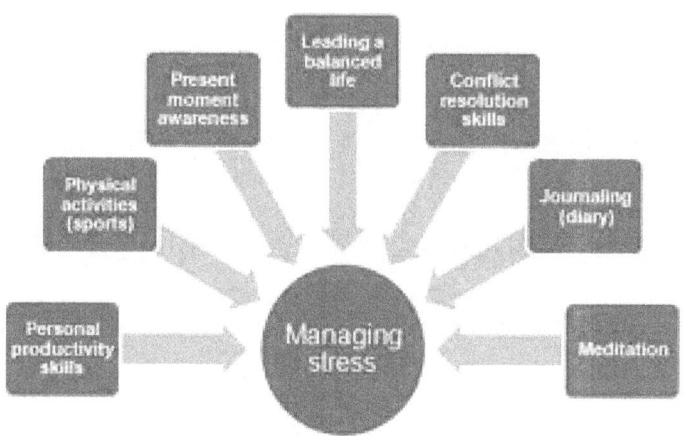

## Manage Stressful People

People can be a major source of stress in our lives. Relatives drive us crazy and co-workers make our jobs harder. Follow this "How To" to reduce the impact stressful people have on your life and your health.

**Difficulty:** Easy
**Time required:** varies

**Here's How:**

1. **Pre-decide**

   You have dealt with this person before, you can probably play the situation out in your head, and you know exactly what they are going do -- so decide what you are going to do. Decide beforehand what you want to do and stick to that.

## 2. **Control Your Reaction**

A person who doesn't care has a tremendous power. If someone upsets you because of what they believe, ask yourself "Why do I care?" You can't change or control people, but you can control how you react to them.

## 3. **Don't Get on Their Emotional Bus**

Stressful people will try to take you on an emotional ride with them. They get angry, you get angry and yelling happens. They get sad, you get sad and everybody's sad. Don't get on their emotional bus. Listen, talk, communicate -- but don't let them control you by triggering negative emotions.

## 4. **Know What You Need**

When meeting with a stressful person, know beforehand what you need from the meeting. What are your goals? Keep those in mind as the conversation ebbs and flows. Bring the talk back to your goals. If you can get your goals met you have learned how to deal with this person.

## 5. **Don't Dwell**

After your encounter with the stressful, don't keep thinking about it. If things went badly, move on with your life. You can be sure the stressful person isn't thinking about you. Don't ruin the rest of your day. Create a plan for next time you are in that situation and let it go.

**Learn To Relax**

Herbert Benson and his group at the <u>Mind-Body Medical Institute</u> have been studying the relaxation response since the 1970s and have linked its use to reductions in high blood pressure. The idea is simple: just as the body responds to certain cues and situations with a stress response, it can also respond a relaxation response. With 20 minutes a day, you can learn to use the relaxation response to reduce stress and to improve blood pressure.

**Difficulty:** Easy
**Time required:** 20 minutes a day

**Here's How:**

1. **Sit**

   Find a comfortable place to sit. Sit with you back straight and feet on the floor. Be comfortable, but alert.

2. **Close your eyes**

   Just relax. Close your eyes. Let everything fall away.

34

### 3. Breathe in

Breathe in through your nose. Feel the breath fill your body.

### 4. Breathe out

Exhale through your nose. Feel your body collapse. Breathe out fully.

### 5. Repeat

Continue breathing. After each time your breath in and out, say (or think) the word "One". Continue for 20 minutes. You can change the word to anything meaningful for you.

### 6. Practice daily

Repeat this every day. Have a set time to do it. Don't worry about setting an alarm; just have a clock nearby that you can see. If you start drifting in thought, gently return to your breathing.

### 7. Mini-relaxations

During your day, stop a few times and 'do a mini'. Just breathe in and out for about a minute. This will relax you and begin to teach your body how to respond to stress in a calm way.

## What You Need

- Place to sit
- 20 uninterrupted minutes

**Think Positive, Live Longer**

Research shows that how you perceive aging affects how long you will live. In a study of 660 people, those with more positive perceptions of their own aging lived an average of 7.5 years longer. This effect remained after other factors such as age, gender, income; loneliness and health status were controlled.

**Look Forward to Aging While You Are Young:**

The study compared death rates of the 660 study participants to their answers to a survey 23 years ago. Therefore, adjusting your perception of aging while you're still young can have a tremendous effect on your life expectancy.

**Improving Resiliency:**

No one knows for sure why a positive attitude seems to lead to a longer life. Researchers believe that positive thinking about aging can increase a person's will to live, making him or her more resilient to illness and more proactive about health. Another explanation given was that mental stress of aging is lower for people who have a positive attitude. Positive thinking and stress reduction have also been linked.

**Finding Insight as You Age:**

What's so great about aging? Good question. Our society prizes youth and beauty above all. Messages about aging tend to emphasize the negative aspects. But, like fine wine, people should get better as they age. Experience, combined with maturity, gives older people great insight. Older people are more in touch with spirituality and the priorities which have true depth. By following a simple, healthy lifestyle you can preserve your health and energy your whole life.

### How Positive Attitudes Compare to Other Longevity Boosters:

Here is a brief list of the number of years that each of these health factors is believed to add (remember these numbers are for mortality and do not consider the quality of life):

- low blood pressure: 4 years
- low cholesterol readings: 4 years
- healthy weight: 1-3 years
- not smoking: 14 years
- regular exercise: 1-3 years

### Worriers Die Younger

Relaxation is good for your health. Every time you worry, feel anxiety or overreact you could be shortening your life. Instead, like good wine, try to mellow with age. As you get older, react to things with patients. This could increase your life expectancy.

A study of over 1,600 men, aged 43 to 91, was conducted to examine how "neurotic" men did over time. The researchers used a personality test and defined a "neurotic personality" as someone who worries too much, feels anxiety or depression and reacts to stress negatively.

The researchers followed the men for 12 years.

The researchers looked at how the "neurotic personality" changed over time. They compared men who were either highly neurotic or who increased in neuroticism over time to men who were mildly neurotic or decreased in neuroticism over time.

At the end of the study, only 50% of the men with high or increasing neuroticism were alive compared to 75-85% of the other group.

Even a small increase in neuroticism over the course of the study led to a 40% increase in death compared to a stable person.

The data was controlled for age and a number of other conditions.

**Why Does Neuroticism Impact Life Expectancy?**
The data can't answer the "why" question. There are a couple of theories that jump to mind – the first is stress. Neurotic people are likely to have more stress hormones in their bodies, causing all sorts of problems and complications. The other is that the lack of positive thinking may impact mortality. Future studies will look at the cortisol level of men (a measure of stress) and negative coping behaviors like smoking.

Whatever the case, if you feel that you are highly neurotic or increasing in neuroticism as you age, consider learning stress reduction and relaxation techniques to increase your longevity. Start with breathing techniques, yoga or simple meditation.

## Chapter 4 - Relationships and Aging

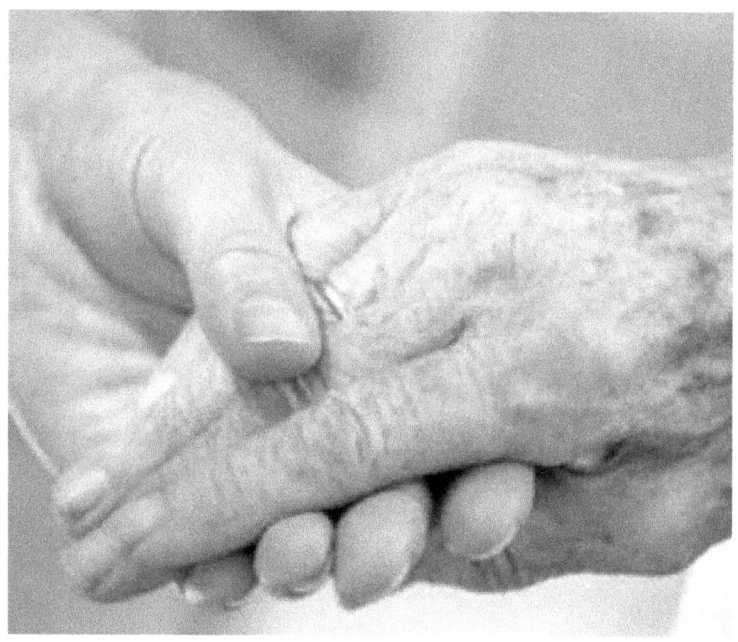

## Avoid Bad Relationships

You may have read somewhere that relationships are good for your health, longevity and life expectancy. In general that's true, except when it's not.

## Bad Relationships Are Bad For Your Health

Anyone who has been through an ugly divorce, difficult parents (or children) or psycho friends can tell you in a second that not all relationships are good for your health.

We all have some people in our lives that create stress and problems (no names, please).

Researchers were able to measure relationship quality in a study of 9,000 men and women in the British civil service. The participants were given surveys about their relationships and the number and type of negative aspects in their close relationships. They were also closely monitored for health problems.

People with more negative aspects in their close relationships had a 34% increase in the risk of heart problems (even after taking weight, social support and other factors into consideration). That's a pretty substantial increase.

## Conclusion

Interacting with most of your friends and family members is a good thing. It increases your life expectancy, protects your brain and more. But interacting with some of your other friends and family members (you know who I'm talking about) can actually make you less healthy. Do your best to maximize the first type of interactions while minimizing the second. You can do this by avoiding the people who are negative in your life, using relaxation techniques to help you "let go" of stress after encountering these people and learning to manage these people actively so they do not impact your life and your health as much. You may have read somewhere (perhaps on the site) that relationships are good for your health, longevity and life expectancy. In general that's true, except when it's not.

## Conclusion

Interacting with most of your friends and family members is a good thing. It increases your life expectancy, protects your brain and more. But interacting with some of your other friends and family members (you know who I'm talking about) can actually make you less healthy. Do your best to maximize the first type of interactions while minimizing the second. You can do this by avoiding the people who are negative in your life, using relaxation techniques to help you "let go" of stress after encountering these people and learning to manage these people actively so they do not impact your life and your health as much.

## Good Relationships Increase Life Expectancy

Relationships are an essential part of health. Isolation and loneliness create responses in the body similar to those of stress. The body does not function as well as when we are connected to other people. Invest time with family and friends not only for happiness, but for physical health too.

## Relationships Help Your Immune System:

Researchers recruited a healthy group of nurses under the age 65 and tested their blood's immune function in correlation with their attachment style in the study. Women with an insecure attachment style had lower immune activity and were more prone to some illnesses. While the link between attachment style and immune function is new, insecure relationships can likely reduce the effectiveness of the immune system through increased stress.

## Perceived Usefulness to Friends and Families is Important for Health:

The MacArthur Study of Successful Aging asked adults aged 70 to 79 how they rate their own usefulness to family and friends. After 7 years, these same people were examined for mortality and other health data. Researchers learned that people who rated their own usefulness high were less likely to suffer from chronic illness or mortality. These findings held true after gender, health, lifestyle and other factors were considered.

Loneliness and the risk of Alzheimer's disease were studied in 823 senior citizens in Chicago. Each person rated their level of loneliness each year for five years. The higher the loneliness rating, the more likely the person would develop cognitive problems during the study. The loneliest 10 percent were more than twice as likely to develop Alzheimer's disease. All results were controlled for measures of actual social contact. This means that what matters is whether a person feels lonely or not, regardless of what kinds of connections he or she has with other people.

## Relationships and Aging

Relationships are an essential part of health. Isolation and loneliness create responses in the body similar to those of stress. The body does not function as well as when we are connected to other people. Invest time with family and friends not only for happiness, but for physical health too.

## Chapter 5 - Emotional and Mental Health

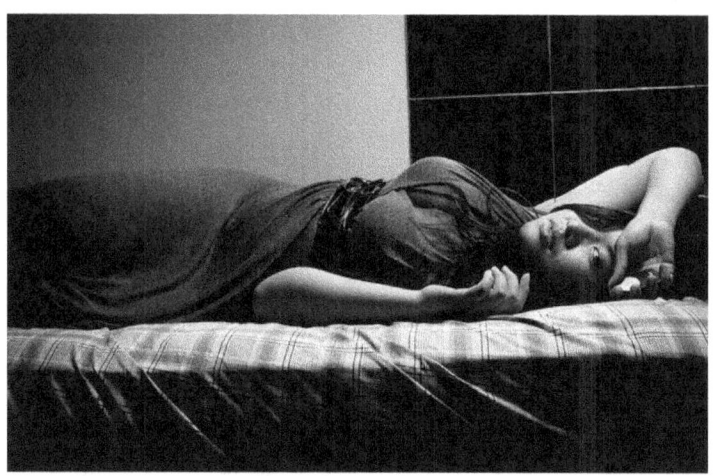

## Vitamin D and Depression

Vitamin D deficiency is being linked with bone trouble, lower back pain, heart trouble and now depression. Linking vitamin D deficiency and depression makes a certain intuitive sense to me.

Vitamin D is produced in your body when your skin is exposed to light.

During winter, many people suffer from seasonal affective disorder (SAD) because of lack of exposure to sunlight.

It kind of makes sense to me that there would be a link between vitamin D deficiency and depression (though, as we will see, researchers aren't certain if vitamin D deficiency causes depression or is a result of depression).

## Vitamin D Deficiency in Older Adults

Over 1,200 men and women between the ages of 65 to 95 were participating in a long-term study of aging. As part of that study, they had extensive blood work done include vitamin D levels. Turned out that about 40% of the men and 57% of the women had vitamin D deficiency.

## Vitamin D Deficiency and Depression

Of all the people in the study, 169 were suffering from minor depression and 26 from major depression. On average, those suffering from depression had vitamin D levels about 14% lower than the others in the study.

Now it gets a bit more complicated. The level of a hormone called parathyroid hormone was elevated in those with depression –- 5% higher in the case of minor depression and 33% higher for those with major depression. Parathyroid hormone often increases as vitamin D levels decrease.

## Could Vitamin D Deficiency Cause Depression?

It could, we just don't know for sure. It could also be true that depression causes low vitamin D levels. There could also be something more complicated going on. If vitamin D deficiency caused depression, that would be fantastic news because vitamin D deficiency is easy to treat with increased exposure to sunlight and supplementation.

## Mental Health as Anti-Aging

Mental health as a strong sense of meaning in your life can be an anti-aging technique. Seniors ages 70 to 78 were asked how useful they felt to others. The more useful they felt, the lower their age-related disability and mortality over a 7-year period. This was true even after health status, age and other factors were considered.

## Be useful

Volunteering is one of the best ways to feel more useful. Find an organization that needs volunteers, or just volunteer to help out a family member or neighbor. Other great ways of being useful are tutoring, mentoring younger people, giving advice based on your experience and teaching your skills, such as cooking or woodworking. Whatever you do, find a way to get involved and feel more useful.

## Statins and Alzheimer's Risk

Researchers report in a 2007 study that statin drugs may prevent brain damage that causes Alzheimer's disease. Statins drugs, widely prescribed for their cholesterol lowering benefits, may protect the brain as well as the heart.

In the study, researchers examined the brains of 110 people aged 65 to 79. They found that the brains of people who had been taking statin drugs had fewer signs of the type of damage (such as plaques and tangles) commonly seen in Alzheimer's disease.

Population-based studies have shown a connection between statins and a reduced risk of Alzheimer's disease before, but this was the first study to examine actual brains of people and find evidence of differences in plaques and other physical signs of Alzheimer's disease based on whether or not people took statins.

## The Conclusion

Since no one knows the causes of Alzheimer's disease, it is difficult to know the full implications of this study. It seems that there is a link between cholesterol, inflammation and an increased risk of Alzheimer's disease. Statin drugs certainly reduce cholesterol and may reduce inflammation. This study gives yet another reason (in addition to preventing heart attacks) for people with high cholesterol to take, and continue taking, statin medications while making lifestyle changes to further reduce cholesterol and inflammation.

## I Have a Special Gift for My Readers

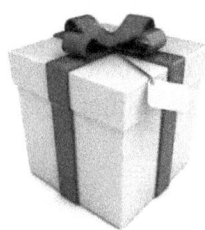

I appreciate my readers for without them I am just another author attempting to make a difference. If my book has made a favorable impression please leave me an honest review. Thank you in advance for you participation.

My readers and I have in common a passion for the written word as well as the desire to learn and grow from books.

My special offer to you is a massive ebook library that I have compiled over the years. It contains hundreds of fiction and non-fiction ebooks in Adobe Acrobat PDF format as well as the Greek classics and old literary classics too.

In fact, this library is so massive to completely download the entire library will require over 5 GBs open on your desktop.

Use the link below and scan all of the ebooks in the library. You can select the ebooks you want individually or download the entire library.

The link below does not expire after a given time period so you are free to return for more books rather than clog your desktop. And feel free to give the link to your friends who enjoy reading too.

I thank you for reading my book and hope if you are pleased that you will leave me an honest review so that I can improve my work and or write books that appeal to your interests.

Okay, here is the link…

http://tinyurl.com/special-readers-promo

PS: If you wish to reach me personally for any reason you may simply write to mailto:support@epubwealth.com.

I answer all of my emails so rest assured I will respond.

**Meet the Author**

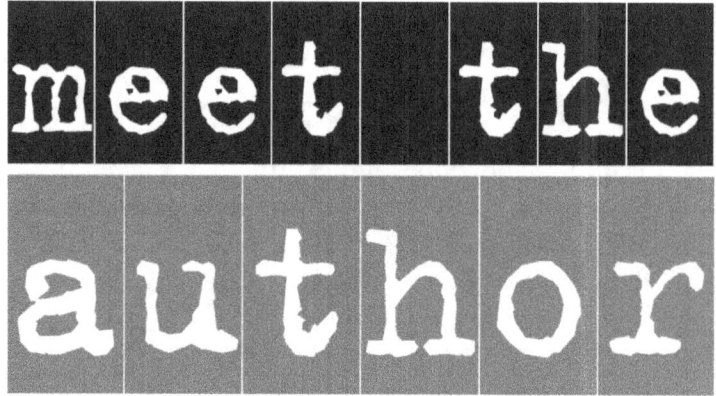

Dr. Noah Pranksky is a research behavioral scientist for Applied Mind Sciences. His research involves many aspects of the human mind including relationships, energy psychology, and various protocols and modalities relating to treatment and cure of various mental maladies.

He and his wife Marianne reside in Portland, Oregon.

**Visit some of his websites**
http://www.AddMeInNow.com
http://www.AppliedMindSciences.com
http://www.AppliedWebInfo.com
http://www.BookbuilderPLUS.com
http://www.BookJumping.com
http://www.EmailNations.com
http://www.EmbarrassingProblemsFix.com
http://www.ePubWealth.com
http://www.ForensicsNation.com
http://www.ForensicsNationStore.com
http://www.FreebiesNation.com
http://www.HealthFitnessWellnessNation.com
http://www.Neternatives.com
http://www.PrivacyNations.com
http://www.RetireWithoutMoney.org
http://www.SurvivalNations.com
http://www.TheBentonKitchen.com
http://www.Theolegions.org
http://www.VideoBookbuilder.com